Coconut Oil Weight Loss

Healthy Long Lasting Fat Loss Without Starving

By

I0426129

Jonas Lee

Coconut oil weight loss is about *healthy weight loss* and *healthy fat loss* using coconut oil! If you are *skeptical* about whether coconut oil can really help you lose weight, please read on. If you think that coconut oil is fattening, you have been misinformed. If you think that coconut oil is bad, then you have been misled.

I don't blame you for your skepticism and disbelief as you have based your information on heresay or some unsubstantiated articles you had read on the internet, such as:

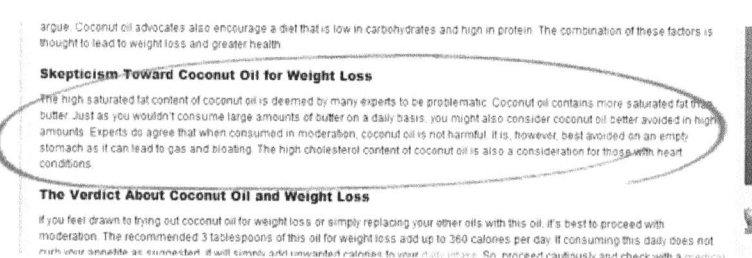

Or

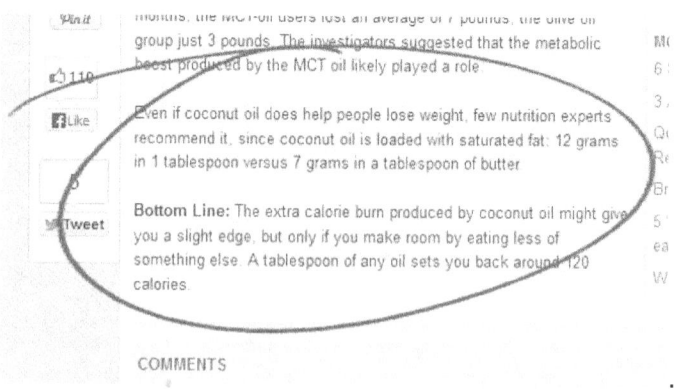

The author is deeply disturbed by health blog writers, including some doctors and nutritionists, who made irresponsible statements about coconut oil without justification.

If you have come across statements that hinted, implied or outright slammed coconut oil as bad because it is a saturated fat, then the people who made those statements were either too lazy to learn about saturated oils or too hurried to finish some article deadlines and not bother to differentiate the types of saturated fats!

In this eBook the author sets out to present his arguments based on research studies and logical interpretation on how and why coconut oil can and will contribute to healthy weight loss. Some of the benefits from reading this eBook are:

- Why should some individuals lose weight while others should not even consider weight loss
- How do you determine you should consider losing some weight
- Know the dangers of quick weight loss
- True weight loss
- How does our body lose weight
- What really is coconut oil
- What are the differences between short-chain, medium-chain, and long-chain fatty acids
- Is coconut oil fattening
- Why are vegetable oils fattening
- Does coconut oil increase your metabolism
- Why isn't coconut oil not stored as fats
- How to take coconut oil

- How much coconut oil should you take

Find out the truth about coconut oil and weight loss in this book.

TABLE OF CONTENTS

Disclaimer

The material in the Coconut Oil Weight Loss eBook is provided for educational and informational purposes only and is not intended as medical advice. The information contained herein should not be used to diagnose or treat any illness, metabolic disorder, diseases or health problem. Always consult your physician or health care provider before beginning any nutrition or exercise program. Use of the programs, advice, and information contained in this eBook is at the sole decision, discretion and risk of the reader.

The author has made his best effort to ensure the information presented to be as accurate as possible. Any health claims presented are based on literature research and scientific reasoning, with interpretation of the author as well as the understanding of the author of other experts' work.

If you have any illness, chronic or otherwise, including diabetes, chronic hypertension, high blood cholesterol, cardiovascular disease, or any other medical condition or metabolic disorder requiring special nutritional considerations, the author suggests you consult a health care professional.

The author and publisher shall have neither liability nor responsibility to any person or entity with respect to any of the information contained in this book/e-book. The user assumes all risk for any injury, loss or damage caused or alleged to be caused, directly or indirectly by using any information described in this program and book.

Introduction

Thank You for purchasing 'Coconut Oil Weight Loss – Healthy & Long Lasting Fat Loss Without Starving'.

Why Coconut Oil Weight Loss?

Whenever I ask my friends, family members, and acquaintances about their views on coconut oil, at least 9 out of 10 people will tell me coconut oil is fattening or coconut oil is bad. Likewise, many doctors, nutritionists and health professionals are still preaching the message that coconut oil is fattening and bad for the heart because it is saturated fat.

Many Doctors, Health Professionals and Nutritionists Are Ignorant of Coconut Oil Research Findings

What deeply saddens me is that the health and medical professionals did not even back their views of coconut oil with any research studies. They either divert the topic or insist that it is the universal truth and 'everybody knows that'.

If you are new to the topic of coconut oil, or if you have been informed that there is no way coconut oil will help you lose weight, this book will provide you with information which your doctor, health professionals and nutritionist would not bother to explain to you in details. Maybe they don't know the answer. Or, maybe they don't care.

Coconut Oil is Better Than Olive Oil!

The astonishing truth is there are scientific studies which demonstrate why coconut oil is better than the other edible oils in helping the body to lose weight healthily. You will be surprised to find that coconut oil is even better than the most glorified and healthiest oil in weight loss effect. That oil is none other than olive oil. We will discuss this in details later in the book.

Watch What You Read on the Internet

I am really annoyed and mad when I read something like the one shown below on the internet. What made it worse was the article was written by a certified dietitian.

Does coconut oil promote weight loss?

As with any fat, coconut oil contains a large amount of calories per gram and is therefore very energy dense. This means that excessive consumption is likely to lead to weight gain.

It has been theorized that the medium chain fatty acids found in coconut oil are more easily burnt than longer fatty acids, but there is no evidence to support the claim that this can aid weight loss or enhance fat burning in the body.

One small study did find that supplementation with coconut oil rather than alternative fats resulted in a modest reduction in waist circumference, but no effects were seen on BMI or fat mass.

Many studies into the effect of medium chain fatty acids have been extrapolated to coconut oil, despite significant difference in composition. Further investigation is required to find out exactly how the combination of fats in coconut oil behaves in the human body.

For those who cannot view the above diagram. It says,
"One small study did find that supplementation with coconut oil rather than alternative fats resulted in modest reduction in waist circumference, but no effects were seen on BMI or fat mass."

There are many more such writings on the internet that reflect either ignorance or irresponsible attitude in making unsubstantiated statements. The major problem with information like the one above is that most people without the technical knowledge will take them as truth. What makes it worse is some of the writings come from some of the largest, reputable health or medical websites.

Purpose of this Book

The purpose of this book is to dispel the notion that coconut oil is fattening. In addition, the book will present the evidence and arguments that not only coconut oil is not fattening, but it is conducive to weight loss. This book will help you understand why and how coconut oil, being a different type of fats, will help you lose weight.

The book will not be complete without knowing how to differentiate good and inferior coconut oil products. For entertainment purposes, I have also thrown in a chapter on celebrities who use coconut oil.

I have included some relevant information in the appendices for those who are uncertain whether they should or when they should lose weight, and also information on how our body loses weight and what healthy weight loss is.

Download Virgin Coconut Oil and Coconut Oil Overview

Finally, I have done up a sheet which lists the main points on coconut oil and virgin coconut oil. It looks like the following picture which you may or may not be able to view in your Kindle.

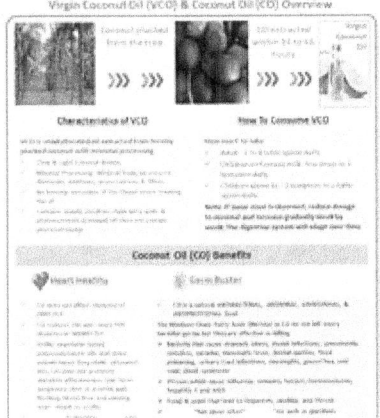

You can download it at http://healthybodytips.org/cowl/. All you need to do is to enter your name and email, and I will email you the download link for the above 'Virgin Coconut Oil and Coconut Oil Overview' as PDF. In the same email, you will also be able to download another pdf named 'Diagrams in Coconut Oil WeightLoss' with all the pictures, charts and photos used in the book for those of you who could not view them in their Kindle.

With that, let's begin our journey together to explore this wonderful topic of Coconut Oil Weight Loss.

Sincerely,
Jonas Lee

Chapter 1. Unintentional testimonials – My Wife & I

"Society is always taken by surprise at any new example of common sense."
Ralph Waldo Emerson

This chapter was not in the book when I first published it. As I was re-structuring and rewriting the book based on readers' feedback, I thought this might be a good time to include our testimonials as an opener for the subject of this book.

Some Background Information

Though I have known the goodness of coconut oil and virgin coconut oil for quite some time, I have not been taking it as a supplement (by the spoonful) until about 2 months ago.

My son (5 years old) was the first person in the family to be on virgin coconut oil. We put him on coconut oil because he was infected with '**hand, foot and mouth disease**'. And shortly after that, my wife also started taking virgin coconut oil. It was around that time we replaced our edible oil with coconut oil. (We had been on canola oil and some olive oil for as long as we could remember.)

At that time I also took coconut oil for a brief period because I had an onset of **shingles** (Varicella Zoster). The virgin coconut oil healed both of my son and me from our conditions. My son's hand, foot and mouth disease was confirmed clinically by a child specialist while mine was self-diagnosed.

(The antimicrobial power of coconut oil is another exciting topic which I am working on in an upcoming book.)

My Weight Loss

First of all, I did not take coconut oil because of overweight or obesity. I was happy with my weight. With a height of 5 feet 9 inches, my weight was about 71kg for a long time, probably for more than a year. That gave me a BMI=23, which falls within the normal weight range. (Please refer to the 2 diagrams below)

I decided to take coconut oil consistently since about 2, 3 months ago. I wanted to know what it would do to my body or health if I were to take it as a supplement by the spoonful. I was not thinking about my weight at all when I decided to take it. My effort lasted about 2 months quite consistently by taking about 1 table spoon a day and sometimes only in my coffee. As far as I know, there was no change in my diet during that period. And I was not on other health supplements (I am the lazy type).

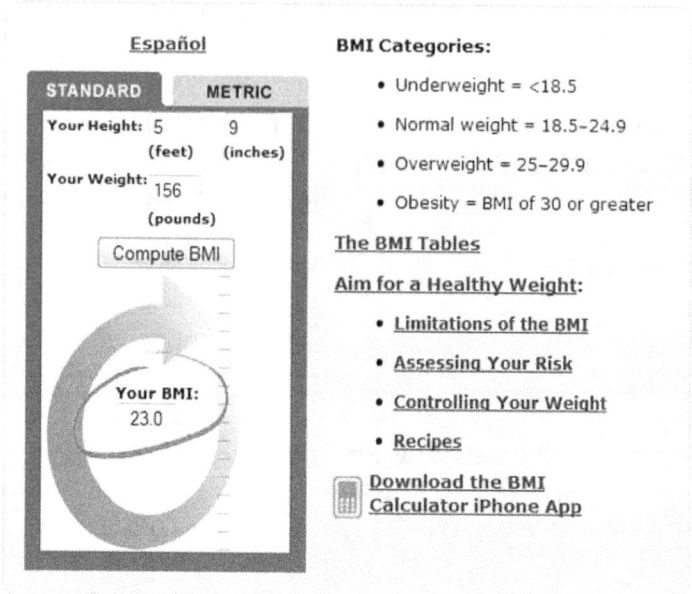

(Source:
http://www.nhlbi.nih.gov/guidelines/obesity/BMI/bmicalc
.htm)

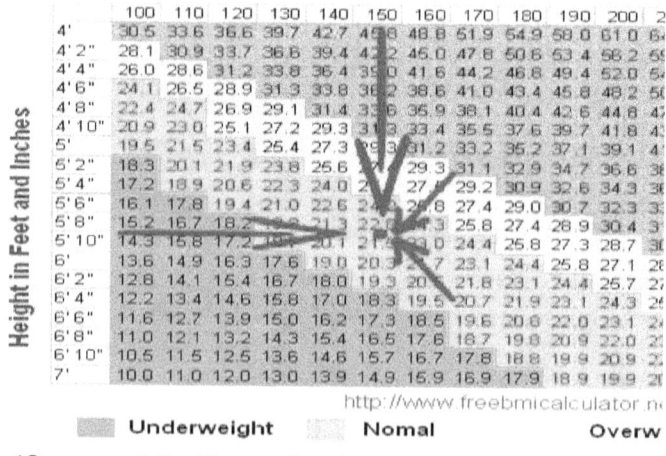

(Source: http://www.freebmicalculator.net/bmi-
chart.php)

Recently, when I weighed myself while we were checking our son's weight, I was weighing 68kg. That caught my attention. The significance of this 'incidental' drop in my weight is NOT the amount of weight lost which was only 3kg (6.6lb). What surprised me was the sudden weight loss after having a consistent weight of 71kg for a long time.

The answer had to be the coconut oil since that was the only change in my diet during that time. And what made it even more convincing was I hadn't exercise for years (lazy type, not good!). It would be interesting to know what would happen if I were to pick up exercise again.

My Wife Gained Weight!

Another surprise was the increase in weight for my wife. For at least 4 years since our child was born, she has been weighing 42kg to 43kg. I always said my wife is too 'skinny' and I wish I could help her gain some weight. Recently, when she stepped onto the weighing scale, the needle peaked at 47kg. We could not quite believe our eyes that she had to weigh herself 3 times to confirm her weight gain. She was on coconut oil for about 3 months. Isn't that marvelous?

Coconut Oil Helps Attain Optimal Weight?

Dr. Bruce Fife did mention in his book 'The Coconut Oil Miracle' that some of his lean readers did observe weight increase by taking coconut oil. **Dr Mary Enig** also mentioned there is a normalization of body lipids (fats) when we take coconut oil.

It is interesting to observe that my weight came down slightly while my wife gained some weight. It is quite logical to think that by consuming coconut oil the overweight person may reduce in weight while the underweight may pick up some weight. In other words, there could be a balancing effect in helping a person attain optimal weight.

With that let's get into the topic of this book – Weight Loss and Coconut Oil.

Chapter 2. Why Coconut Oil Is Not Fattening

"Recently published research has shown that natural coconut fat in the diet leads to a normalization of body lipids, protects against alcohol damage to the liver, and improves the immune system's anti-inflammatory response. Clearly, there has been increasing recognition of health-supporting functions of the fatty acids found in coconut" – Mary Enig Ph.D., F.A.C.N.

Technical & Fundamental Information

The beginning portion of this presentation may be technical to some readers but it is necessary if we desire to know the truth about coconut oil. The technical details involve understanding the specific types of oils and fats.

Based on the current status of research findings, a meaningful discussion and understanding of edible oils and fats call for a *deeper level of details*. In other words, we can no longer *limit* our discussion to *saturated fat* versus *unsaturated fat* without knowing which particular types of saturated or unsaturated fats we are talking about.

There are many types of saturated fats/oils. Some saturated fats are really bad but some are extremely good. Likewise, a meaningful discussion of unsaturated fats or oils requires differentiation of the specific types. Not all unsaturated fats are equal. Olive oil has long been hailed as healthy because it is monounsaturated, not polyunsaturated or saturated. But, not all monounsaturated oils are good.

Please try to strive through the technical details of this chapter as it is instrumental in understanding why coconut oil is different and good. Here we go.

What are fats?

Fats, as we all know, are *fattening* because they are fats. Basically, that means fats can make us fat. Loosely speaking, all oils are considered to be fats. Fats are also known as **fatty acids**. The term 'Lipid' is another scientific name used to encompass fats, oils, triglycerides, phospholipids and so on.

Fats and oils are often used interchangeably to mean the same thing. However, some refer to fats as solid as in lard and tallow. Others refer to oils as liquid such as canola oil, olive oil, etc.

For our purpose here, oils are fats and fats are oils. Solid fats can melt at a higher temperature and become liquid. Similarly, liquid oil becomes solid when the temperature goes below its melting point.

What happens to fats when they enter our body?

Fats, which we consume from our food, are stored as fats in the body if they are not used or burned as energy. That's why they are regarded as fattening because they make us fat. But, not all fats and oils are equal. Coconut oil is the exception. (We will come to that later)

When fats are stored in the body, they are stored in the form of *triglycerides*. There are many places in our body where fats are stored or deposited. Some are visible on our body while others are within the body.

Some common sites where fat storage is visible include the flaps on our thigh, underarms and the spare tire around the waist.

Fat is one of the 3 macronutrients needed by our body. The other two are *protein* and *carbohydrate*. Carbohydrate and fat have the role of providing *energy* to fuel the functions of our body while protein is broken down into amino acids for building new proteins within the body.

When there isn't enough carbohydrate or fat, protein can also produce energy. When there is too much protein, it can also be converted into fat for storage. *Any fat storage in the body will result in weight gain.* The fat stored can be from excess fat, carbohydrate or protein.

Key point:
>*Any excess fat, carbohydrate and/or protein are stored as fat, resulting in weight gain.*

Fat Storage & Weight Gain Based on Energy or Calorie Analysis

Energy is measured in the form of *calories*. When we consume too much of any of the macronutrients (carbohydrate, protein, or fat), the excess which are not used will be stored as *energy reserves* in the form of *fats*.

These energy reserves are supposed to be used when we do not eat enough to supply the calories needed or when our activities require more energy than the supply from our food intake. This may sound complicated but it's really quite simple.

Example:
> Let's say we need only 3000 calories, but the food we consume provides a total of 3500 calories. The surplus of 500 calories has to be stored, and will be stored as fats. Even if you consume only carbohydrates and/or proteins, but when the total calories exceed the 3000 calories requirements, the extra will still be stored as fats!

Types of Fats in Edible Oils

Edible oils are oils we use for our cooking or food preparation. Edible oils are mostly **vegetable oils**. The term 'vegetable oil' can be misleading because *not all vegetable oils are from vegetables*. Any oils extracted from plant source are considered to be vegetable oils.

Vegetable oils can come from various sources such as seeds, nuts, citrus, melons, etc. Most vegetable oils belong to the major oil crops category while others belong to a large group of minor oil crops.

As such, there are a large number of vegetable oils in the market. A list of *common vegetable oils* is as follows:

- Corn oil
- Soybean oil
- Sunflower oil
- Safflower oil
- Rapeseed/Canola Oil
- Cottonseed oil
- Peanut oil
- Olive oil

- Palm oil
- Coconut oil
- Sesame oil

Vegetable oils essentially consist of triglycerides. In other words, when oil manufacturers extract oil from a plant source, they are extracting the triglycerides.

Triglycerides are nothing more than *3 fatty acids bonded together through a glycerol backbone* (picture below). The 'Tri' accounts for the 3 fatty acid molecules while the 'glyceride' implies the glycerol backbone.

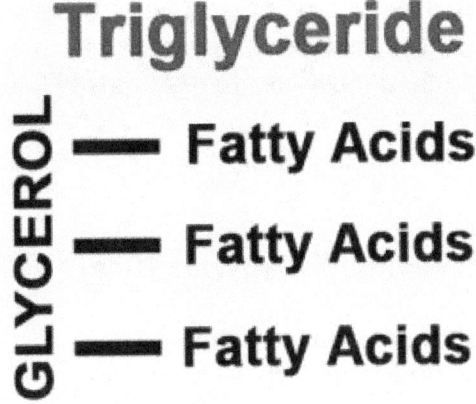

The 3 fatty acids of a triglyceride can take on different types of fatty acids which we will address next.

Types of Fatty Acids

All fatty acids are made up of the same basic structure shown in the diagram below:

Fatty Acids

$$\underset{HO}{\overset{\displaystyle \overset{\text{O}}{\|}}{C}}-C-C-C-$$

Different fatty acids vary in the number of carbons (C) and the number of hydrogen attached to the carbon backbone. These 2 variations will determine the properties and characteristics of a fatty acid.

Naturally occurring fatty acids usually have an even number of carbon atoms, ranging from 4 carbons to 28 carbons. As you can imagine, when you compute the combination between the variations, there can be a large number of fatty acids. Different fatty acids will have different properties and behavior. And , different fatty acids can be found in different vegetable or edible oils.

Top Level Classification of Fatty Acids (Oils)

Based on the extent of saturation of fatty acids, scientists have classified them into 3 major groups:
- Saturated,
- Monounsaturated, and
- Polyunsaturated

When a fatty acid is saturated, it means its carbon atoms are completely filled (or saturated) with hydrogen. Technically, there will be no double bond present. When a fatty acid is unsaturated, its carbon atoms are not completely filled with hydrogen. In other words, there is one or more double bond present in the fatty acid or oil.

Double bond is a weak bond and is subject to oxidation. Oxidation as we all know is not a good thing when it comes to food and health. In fatty acid or oil, they use the technical term peroxidation. But let's not get caught in too much technicality. This is what makes oil rancid.

The key here is saturated fatty acids are not easily oxidized as compared to unsaturated fatty acids. Just this property alone should trigger your mind to ask the question, 'Are unsaturated oils subject to oxidation?' You bet they are.

And the most ridiculous thing is, the process of hydrogenation is used to saturate the oil to reduce the double bonds so that rancidity problem is solved. In other words, the manufacturers will flush the oil with hydrogen to get rid or reduce the double bond so that oxidation is cut to a minimum. Yet the supporters of unsaturated oils keep slamming on how bad saturated oil is! Isn't that ridiculous?

Fatty Acids & Their Sources

A summary of specific fatty acids is shown in the following table for your reference.

No. of Carbons	Name of Fatty Acids	N. of Double Bonds	Source of Fatty Acids	Classification
2	Acetic Acid	0	Vinegar	Saturated
4	Butyric Acid	0	Goat's milk, butter, parmesan cheese	Saturated
6	Caproic Acid	0	Animal fats & oils, gingko, vanilla	Saturated
8	Caprylic Acid	0	Milk, coconut oil, palm kernel oil	Saturated
10	Capric Acid	0	Milk, coconut oil, palm kernel oil	Saturated

12	Lauric Acid	0	Coconut oil, palm kernel oil, laurel oil, human breast milk, goat's milk, cow's milk	Saturated
14	Myristic Acid	0	Nutmeg, coconut oil, palm kernel oil, butter fat	Saturated
16	Palmitic Acid	0	Palm oil, Palm Kernel oil, meats, cheese, dairy products	Saturated
	Palmitoleic Acid	1	Macadamia oil, sea blackthorn oil, animal oils, other vegetable oils	Monounsaturated
18	Stearic Acid	0	Animal fat, vegetable fat, cocoa butter, shea butter	Saturated
	Oleic Acid	1	Olive oil, many animal fats such as turkey fat, chicken fat, and many vegetable oils such as pecan oil, canola oil, etc	Monounsaturated
	Linoleic Acid	2	Many vegetable oils such as poppy seed oil, sunflower oil, safflower oil, corn oil	Polyunsaturated
	Alpha-linolenic Acid	3	Many vegetable oils, chia oil, flaxseed oil, walnut oil	Polyunsaturated
20	Arachidic Acid	0	Peanut oil, corn oil	Saturated
	Arachidonic Acid	4	Peanut oil	Polyunsaturated
	Eicosapentaemoic Acid (EPA)	5	Fish oil, cod liver oil, human breast milk, herring, mackerel, salmon, sardine	Polyunsaturated
22	Erucic Acid	1	Rapeseed/Canola oil, Mustard oil	Monounsaturated
	Docosahexaenoic Acid (DHA)	6	Fish oil, breast milk	Polyunsaturated

Secondary Classification of Fatty Acids (Oils): Short-chain, Medium-chain, and Long-chain Fatty Acids.

The fatty acids listed in the above summary are further classified into 3 different types of acids based on the length of the carbon chain.

Short-chain fatty acids are fats with 2 to 6 carbons. Butyric acid, a short-chain fatty acid, can be found in butter, goat's milk and parmesan cheese. Its structure is shown in the diagram below:

Medium-chain fatty acids are fats with 8 to 12 carbons.
Coconut oil contains 91 to 92% saturated fats, which are primarily medium-chain fatty acids. Palm oil with 50 to 51% saturated fats also has a significant amount of medium-chain fatty acids. Sometimes, the fatty acids with 6 carbons are also considered to be medium-chain.

The 3 most important medium-chain fatty acids in coconut oil are **Caprylic acid**, **Capric acid** and **Lauric acid**. Lauric acid with 12 carbons is shown below:

Long-chain fatty acids are fats with 14 to 24 carbons.

Animal oils and most vegetable oils are primarily long-chain fatty acids. Stearic acid, with 18 carbons, can be found in animal fats such as beef fat and also in many vegetable oils. Its structure is shown below:

$$H-O-\overset{\displaystyle O}{\overset{\|}{C}}-\overset{\displaystyle H}{\underset{\displaystyle H}{\overset{|}{\underset{|}{C}}}}-\overset{\displaystyle H}{\underset{\displaystyle H}{\overset{|}{\underset{|}{C}}}}-\overset{\displaystyle H}{\underset{\displaystyle H}{\overset{|}{\underset{|}{C}}}}-\overset{\displaystyle H}{\underset{\displaystyle H}{\overset{|}{\underset{|}{C}}}}-\cdots-H$$

Coconut Oil is Primarily Medium-chain Fatty Acids

The fats in coconut oil are primarily **medium-chain fatty acids** (MCFAs). The fats in other vegetable oils are mostly **long-chain fatty acids** (LCFAs) and polyunsaturated fats. The metabolism of MCFAs is different from that of LCFAs and polyunsaturated fats.

Another technical term clarification
Strictly speaking, the fats in the coconut oil are in the form of **Medium-Chain Triglycerides** (MCT). You can actually purchase MCT oil in the store. But, once the MCT enters the body, it will be broken down into MCFAs, which can be diglycerides (with 2 fatty acids attached), monoglycerides (with one fatty acid attached), and free fatty acids.

Similarly, the fats in other vegetable oils exist in the form of Long-Chain Triglycerides (LCT). The breakdown of LCT is much more complex than that of MCT..

MCFAs in Coconut Oil are Converted into Energy, Not Fats

The MCFAs contained in Coconut Oil are not absorbed into the villi of the intestines like the LCFAs. Instead, the MCFAs are transported through the hepatic portal vein into the liver, where they are immediately converted into energy instead of fats.

Without being too technical, the MCFAs in coconut oil leave the intestines and enter the liver through the hepatic vein (refer to diagram below). From there, the MCFAs then enter the liver.

The implication of this pathway of transport indicates that MCFAs are absorbed more efficiently compared to LCFAs. The metabolism of MCFAs therefore uses less resources. The MCFAs then enter the mitochondria of the cells where they undergo preferential oxidation to produce energy.

The above statement may be a bit technical but the whole point is MCFAs can be efficiently and quickly be used as energy source without being stored as fats.

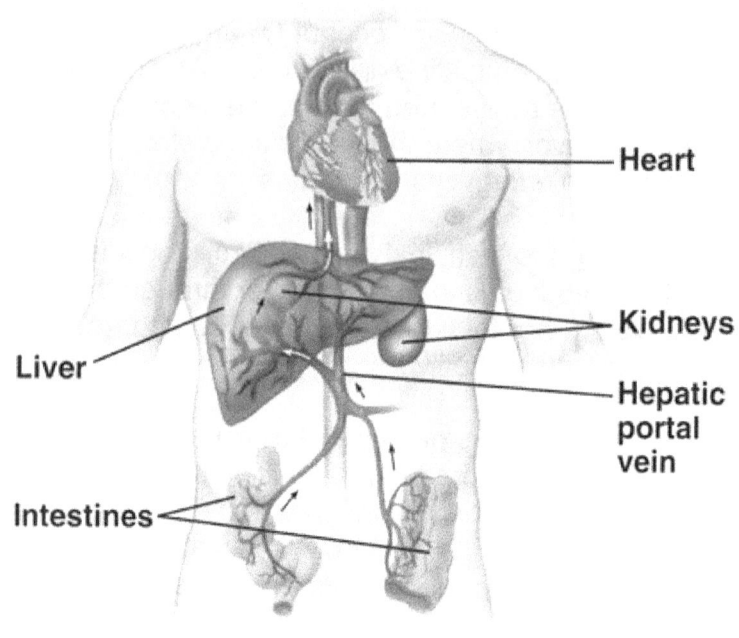

Heart

Kidneys

Liver

Hepatic
portal
vein

Intestines

(Source of diagram:
http://www.lookfordiagnosis.com/mesh_info.php?term=Portal+S
ystem&lang=1)

Coconut Oil is Converted into Energy and Not Stored as Fats –
That's Why Coconut Oil is NOT FATTENING

On the other hand, LCFAs are absorbed into the villi and are then converted into triglycerides (which are essentially fats and the form of fats stored in our body if not fully utilized). These triglycerides are then coated with cholesterol and protein, and subsequently transported through the lymphatic system and then into the bloodstream to be circulated throughout the body.

Important Difference:

The metabolism and pathway of MCFAs and LCFAs set the coconut oil and other vegetable oils apart. MCFAs from coconut oil bypass the form of fats to be stored in the body. LCFAs from other vegetable oils must be in the form of triglycerides which is the form of fats stored in the body (if unutilized).

The actual processes are more complicated than what has been presented here. But the main difference I would like to point out here are:

- LCFAs (as those in vegetable oils) require elaborate modification before they can be transported for body use. MCFAs (as those in Coconut Oil) do not require modification (therefore more efficient) before transportation to site of use
- LCFAs, if unutilized, end up as fats in the body.
- MCFAs are directly converted into energy and not stored as fats.

While both MCFAs and LCFAs are fats and oils, their pathway, metabolism, ultimate fate and forms are different once they enter into the body. As a result, MCFAs and hence Coconut Oil will not contribute to fat storage in your body.

LCFAs, however, and therefore all other vegetable oils will result in fat storage in your body if there is surplus of the oil. This is the critical difference between Coconut Oil and other vegetable oils. Understanding this point alone tells us the ability of Coconut Oil to contribute to weight loss.

Tips on Weight Loss Using Coconut Oil

But weight loss with Coconut Oil will only be realized if you **REPLACE** your edible oil with Coconut Oil. You need to get this point right. *Replacement is the key.*

If you have been using vegetable oils and are still using them in your cooking, then it's unlikely you will see any changes in weight even if you add coconut oil to your diet. Instead, you will likely see increase in weight because the MCFAs will still be burned as energy but the LCFAs from the vegetable oil which you did not replace, will be packaged into more fats (triglycerides) and stored in your body.

In another scenario, if you have replaced your vegetable oil with Coconut Oil, it will be an improvement. But if you increase your consumption of carbohydrates and proteins beyond your normal consumption, you will still see increase in weight. (Remember we mentioned above that any surplus consumption of carbohydrates and/or protein will still end up as fats storage.)

I know I have gone all out trying to make my point clear, or perhaps a bit too much, but I feel this is where either you get it or you don't get it.

Coconut Oil is NOT something that you take and the fats will just go away like magic. That is not going to happen.

The human body is the human body. That is how our body handles different fats, carbohydrates and protein. Once you understand how your body functions and deals with fats and the other 2 macronutrients, consuming MCFAs (Coconut Oil) become the better weight loss choice.

Key Takeaways

- Coconut oil is not fattening because it is converted into energy instead of being stored as fats
- Coconut oil is converted into energy because its fatty acids, primarily medium-chain fatty acids, have a different metabolism than other fatty acids
- Long-chain fatty acids, commonly found in other vegetable oils, are repackaged into triglycerides which will be stored as fats if unutilized.
- Replacing your existing edible oils with coconut oil is the most effective way to help the body lose weight

Chapter 3. 5 Major Reasons Coconut Oil Contributes to Weight Loss

The ability of coconut oil to bring about weight loss boils down to its characteristics. Here, we list 5 major reasons why coconut oil can contribute to weight loss:

1. Coconut oil is not fattening because it is converted into energy and not stored as fats
2. Coconut oil can help burn more fats because it increases the metabolic rate
3. Coconut oil is not fattening because it does not depress thyroid activity and thyroid hormone secretion
4. Coconut oil is not fattening because it has lower calories than all vegetable oils and most edible oils
5. Coconut oil, as with all oils, can make a person feel satiated

The first point has been discussed in the previous chapter. We will now discuss each of the other 4 points.

2. Coconut oil increases metabolic rate.

By increasing the metabolic rate, our body will be able to burn more calories. In other words, higher metabolic rate enables more fats to be burned.

Nutritionists are well aware that the food we eat can influence our **BMR**, or basal metabolic rate. The technical term for this phenomenon is known as diet-induced thermogenesis.

Diet-induced Thermogenesis

Thermogenesis may sound very technical. It is basically the process of heat production in our body. Thermogenesis generally can use up to about 10% (or higher) of the total energy intake from food, depending on the types of food. In other words, thermogenesis actually burns more calories from the food we eat.

Diet-induced thermogenesis is the process of heat production triggered by certain food intake. Essentially when we consume food, cellular activities are stimulated and increased to bring about metabolism.

Protein-rich foods tend to increase thermogenesis more than carbohydrates. This is one of the explanations why high-protein diet results in weight loss (assuming there is no overeating). However, do take note that high protein diet also results in high water loss.

The MCFAs in Coconut Oil can pump up thermogenesis even further, higher than those of high-protein diet. This is incredibly great news for those who want to lose weight.

Many research studies have shown the above characteristics years ago which many proponents of vegetable oils have deliberately ignored.

By comparing the thermogenesis of diets containing MCFAs of LCFAs, study had shown that the calorie-burning effect of MCFAs was almost double that of LCFAs. In other words, **MCFAs can induce the body to burn 2 times more calories than LCFAs**!

Further continuing study also showed that if MCFA-rich diet was taken *continually* for 6 days, a person can end up burning up 50% of the calories from food intake.

Take a minute to absorb this fact – 50% thermogenesis effect! Can you imagine the weight loss effect from 50% more calorie-burning! This is insane but proven beyond a shadow of doubt.

That is not all. Another study, which fed a meal containing 400 calories of MCFAs or 400 Calories of LCFAs, showed that the *thermogenesis of MCFAs over a 6-hour period was 3 times higher than that of LCFAs.*

This study specifically mentioned that the greater MCFAs thermogenesis effect was true as long as there was *no overeating.*

We are not done yet. Another study compared thermogenesis effects of MCFAs in meals for normal-weight versus obese individuals. The results will literally blow your mind away. The study showed that normal-weight persons were burning 48% more calories than if they were eating normal meal, while obese individuals were burning **65%** more calories than their usual meal without MCFAs.

This basically says that if a person has more fats, the MCFAs will pump up the metabolic rate even more than those with less body fats. Isn't this incredible news for people carrying an obese body around?

Key Point
> *The MCFAs from coconut oil will*
> *increase your metabolic rate*
> *better than LCFAs from other*

vegetable oils,
thereby enabling your body to burn
more fats!

3. Coconut oil does not depress thyroid activity and thyroid hormone secretion

Vegetable oils, which are also polyunsaturated fatty acids, have the effect of *depressing thyroid activity*. In other words, polyunsaturated oils *block the secretion of thyroid hormone*, which subsequently leads to *reduced metabolic rate*.

This is more prevalent in excessive consumption of soy, which contains goitrogens. Goitrogens are the antithyroid components in soy which can interfere with the utilization of iodine or functioning of the thyroid gland and cause thyroid problems. They can also reduce the efficiency of thyroid hormone.

The **antithyroid effect** of vegetable oils was first observed in animal farm decades ago. In the 1940s, there was a very famous cow experiment where farmers trying to fatten their cows by feeding them with coconut oil. Unfortunately, the end result was the reverse of what the farmers wanted. The cows fed with coconut oil became lean and active.

In the livestock industry, **antithyroid drug** was used to fatten animals even though they were eating less feed. The problem was antithyroid drug was found to be **carcinogenic** and was likely causing hypothyroidism in people who ate the meat of the animals fed with the antithyroid drug.

They also found that the same anithyroid effect could also be achieved by feeding the animals with *soy and corn feed.* Further experiments showed that animals fed with unsaturated oils were *fattened!*

In essence, **polyunsaturated fat suppresses thyroid activity**, hindering the secretion of thyroid hormone, thus leading to depressed metabolism. That is how **polyunsaturated oils promote weight gain** and why **polyunsaturated vegetable fats are fattening**.

Coconut Oil, on the other hand, does not have any antithyroid effect. Therefore, coconut oil neither depresses the activity of thyroid nor blocks the secretion of thyroid hormone. In addition, Coconut Oil also increases metabolic rate, thus promoting weight loss.

Warning
Polyunsaturated fats from vegetable oils possess antithyroid effect, leading to reduced metabolic rate, thereby promotes weight gain.
Polyunsaturated fats in vegetable oils are FATTENING!

4. Coconut Oil Has Lower Calories

The lower calorie content of Coconut Oil is mentioned here for your information though it does not account for the major weight loss effect of Coconut Oil.

Nevertheless, coconut oil is a few calories lower than polyunsaturated vegetable oils. Most literatures reported that one table spoon (14g) of coconut oil gives 117 calories while that of vegetable oils contains 120 calories or more.

5. Coconut Oil Makes You Feel Satiated

This point is thrown in so you know it does exist. But, this is also applicable to other vegetable oils. Most of us have experienced by consuming more oil, we tend to feel fuller, thereby reducing our food intake. But, because coconut oil is converted into energy, it tends to provide energy better than the other oils. Therefore, the person will feel less need to eat food for energy.

There are studies that demonstrate olive oil is most superior of all oils in making one feel fuller. The studies even indicated that smelling olive oil can have the effect of fullness!

Coconut Oil Versus Olive Oil on Weight Loss & Fat Loss

This subtopic may seem a bit odd as I only choose to discuss olive oil in relation to coconut oil. This is done because many people assume that olive oil is the healthiest, and hence this oil is superior in its properties, functions and effects to all other oils. Below you will see that it may not be true.

In an experiment looking at weight loss program for obese individuals over a 16 week period, the researchers from Columbia University and New York Obesity Research Center studied the effects of MCT oil (which breaks into MCFAs upon consumption) and olive oil on the effect of weight loss.

They discovered that MCT oil induced greater weight loss than olive oil. They also found that MCT oil reduced much more body trunk fat mass, total fat mass and interabdominal adipose tissue than olive oil.

Many people simply assume olive oil is the healthiest oil among the edible oils. While olive oil is still a very good oil (as long as you don't heat it for cooking), the above studies showed that coconut oil is much more superior than olive oil when it comes to weight loss and fat loss.

Controversies and Arguments Against Coconut Oil

Before we close this chapter on coconut oil weight loss, we need to look at several important issues involving why opponents of coconut oil attack the 'claims' on the oil.

I believe it was **Dr Bruce Fife** who wrote that in the scientific world, it is extremely difficult to get funding on coconut oil research. The major reasons for that were mainly due to commercial interests and motives.

We need to interpret things by taking a bigger picture of the edible oil market. In the US, coconut is not grown at all but other edible oils such as canola, corn, sunflower, etc are important oil crops contributing to the US economy and the exporting sector.

Though we can never prove that, do you honestly think that the relevant funding sectors and parties will contribute funds towards research on coconut oil which is grown only in the tropical countries? I think you get the idea and understand what I am trying to say.

Another major problem in funding coconut or coconut oil research is that the research results might not be too welcoming to the pharmaceutical industries. But when it comes to MCT oil, it's a different story.

The pharmaceutical industry makes use of MCT oil. Therefore, there is plenty of research done using MCT oil. (MCT oil consists of caprylic and capric acids with 8 and 10 carbons respectively.)

Coconut oil consists of both caprylic and capric acids. Therefore, some of the research references for coconut oil are drawn from work involving MCT oil. This becomes a loophole for the objection of those who dispute the validity of the claims since actually coconut oil was not used. But, many researches involving MCT actually used MCT extracted from coconut oil.

Key Takeaways

- From the view point of nutrition and scientific evidence, the ability of coconut oil in bringing about weight loss, or rather fat loss, is undeniable and indisputable.
- Coconut oil is effective in weight loss due to the following reasons:
  - ✓ Coconut oil is converted into energy and not stored fats in the body
  - ✓ Coconut oil increases the metabolic rate
  - ✓ Coconut oil does not suppress thyroid functions
  - ✓ Coconut oil has lower calories
- Do keep in mind that when a person overeats or indulges in overeating, nothing will help reduce weight.
- Coconut oil works by replacing your existing edible oil without food indulgence.

- Weight loss results using Coconut Oil will be gradual and healthy. You will likely see loss of a few pounds in a month rather than 10 pounds in a week or two. And the few pounds of weight loss using Coconut Oil will never damage or cause harm to your health.

Chapter 4. Coconut Oil Versus Virgin Coconut Oil

Coconut oil is different from virgin coconut oil. The difference between the two boils down to the manufacturing processes.

Virgin coconut oil (VCO) is a coconut oil with minimal processing and is as unadulterated as possible. Most VCOs are produced with minimal heat, no chemicals, and no enzymes. Therefore, VCO also contains valuable phytonutrients in addition to the medium-chain triglycerides.

Coconut oil, on the other hand, has gone through more processing compared to VCO. Coconut oil is often called copra or RBD oil, where RBD stands for refined, bleached and deodorized. Copra is basically dried coconut meat. Therefore, oil extracted from copra has to undergo refining, bleaching and bleaching before it is edible. Nevertheless, the medium-chain fatty acids are still present in coconut oil.

Key Point:
> *Medium chain triglycerides are present in both coconut oil and virgin coconut oil. However, important phytonutrients are no longer retained in coconut oil due to its processing.*

For cooking purposes, it is more economical to use coconut oil. For use as dietary supplement (eating by the spoonful), virgin coconut oil is recommended.

Brands of Coconut Oil & Virgin Coconut Oil

There are many brands of coconut oil and virgin coconut oil in the market. You need to shop around where you live. In my part of the world, Malaysia, I normally find them in pharmacy and organic store. You can also find them online, Amazon and other individual sites.

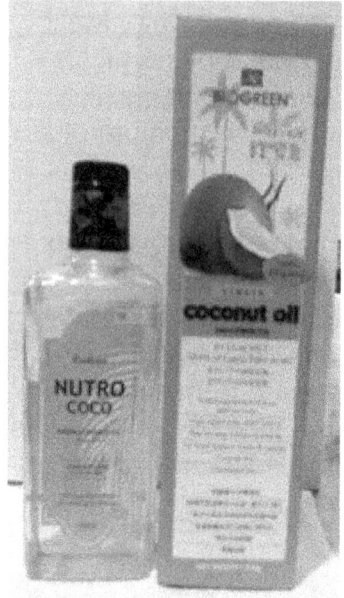

The above photo shows two of the brands of VCO my family is taking. Both are decent quality VCOs which fit the criteria I discuss in the following section.

Let me make this clear. I am neither promoting any brand nor am I an agent of any brand (may be one day but I will let you know if I do become one).

I know of one superior quality brand (pricey in Malaysia) which you can purchase online. The brand is

COCOLAB. The owner is a coconut oil scientist in Malaysia. He is a specialist in coconut oil and I have learned so much from him. He gets a lot of order from outside of Malaysia. He told me the delivery charges to some overseas countries are much more than the product cost but still people are buying from his website.

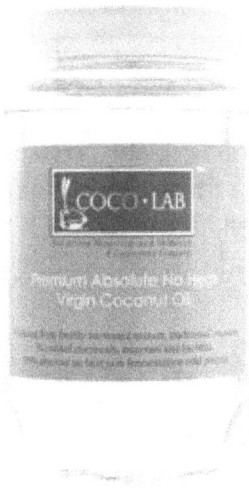

He has a whole range of coconut oil products, ranging from dietary supplement to skin care. You can check it out at http://www.cocolab.my/. You can contact him and you may mention me but I am not promising or promoting any special deal (he doesn't even know I am talking about him or his products here. His name is Alex.)

Though I cannot advise you on the brands other than the above because the brands that I use are likely not available in your local stores (and the brand you can find may not be available here), I urge you to read the next section on how to differentiate the quality of coconut oil.

Buying Quality Virgin Coconut Oil

Good quality virgin coconut oil should be colorless with a light coconut aroma. When it is in the liquid form, it should be crystal clear. When you put a good quality VCO in the refrigerator, the color should be as white as snow.

Another characteristic of quality virgin coconut oil is the absence of burning sensation at the throat when taken by the spoonful. It's quite easy to tell if you have 2 different brands in front of you. Good quality VCO is smooth to swallow without any burning or mild 'spicy-like' feel when it passes through your throat. You really need to try it to know it.

Some VCOs have a yellowish tint which is inferior to those of colorless. If the VCO has a yellowish tint to it, its quality is not the best. The yellowish tint is a sign of mishandling during processing, due to contamination (molding or residue) or overheating.

In addition, VCOs with strong coconut taste and aroma are likely to be more processed than those of light flavor and aroma.

VCOs labeled with 'Extra' are purely marketing gimmicks without any difference in quality from any good VCO. Unlike Olive oil, virgin coconut oil has no international or agreed standard criteria that define one to be 'extra'.

Key Takeaways

- Virgin Coconut Oil is a coconut oil with minimal amount of processing compared to coconut oil which has been subject to refining, bleaching and deodorization
- Coconut oil is also void of the phytonutrients present in Virgin Coconut Oil
- Quality Virgin Coconut Oil is characterized by colorless and light coconut flavour and aroma; it will not produce a burning sensation at the throat when taken by the spoonful

Chapter 5. How To Take Coconut Oil

Taking Coconut Oil as Dietary Supplement

There are many ways you can take coconut oil. The best option would be to take it as a supplement. In other words, pour the oil into a table spoon and take it as such. In this case, Virgin Coconut Oil is recommended as it contains also phytonutrients.

Unfortunately, not everybody can take coconut oil or virgin coconut oil as is. I personally find it tasty and delicious. However, some people do not like the feel or idea of eating oil!

If you are unable to swallow coconut oil by the spoonful, there are many ways you can incorporate into your daily schedule.

You can mix a spoonful of the oil in your coffee, tea, soup, or your favorite beverages. I use it in my coffee in addition to taking it by the spoonful.

You can also pour the oil onto rice, cereals, mashed potatoes, noodles, or porridge. The oil can also be used as salad dressing, sauce, bread spread or bread dip. I can imagine it might be a problem to use it as salad dressing in the winter. I am in a tropical country so I can't really tell you how you could do it without having a warm or hot salad.

The limit is really up to your imagination. Just treat it like your normal edible oil.

Coconut Oil in Cooking

As we discussed in the chapter on coconut oil weight loss, the best effect is to replace all your edible oil with coconut oil. If you want to do that, it is better to use copra or RBD coconut oil, not virgin coconut oil.

First, it is wasteful to heat up virgin coconut oil for cooking. Second, the phytonutrients will likely be lost on heating. Third, it is also more economical because you may use more oil for cooking than if you were to take the oil by the spoonful.

How Much Should I Take?

It is generally recommended to take around 3 table spoons per day. You don't have to take it all in one go. You can split up the portion throughout the day.

You will find some conflicting opinion on the daily portion of coconut oil and virgin coconut oil on the internet. Most, if not all, of those who advise taking a table spoon or sparingly are the ones who have no experience in using the oil. Many of these are doctors, nutritionists, and health professionals.

As recommended by **Dr Bruce Fife**, the author of The Coconut Oil Miracle, take the oil for at least 3 months before you conclude whether it works. (Please read the possible reaction section below)

For Weight Loss Purpose

If you are taking it for weight loss purposes, the best effect will be to replace all your edible oil with coconut oil. Because it is used as a food and edible oil in your daily food preparation and cooking, do not coconut oil to be like magic weight loss pill.

The weight loss will be gradual over the course of weeks to months before you realize it. This method of coconut oil weight loss is healthy while reaping the benefits of shedding unhealthy fats. So, do not expect to see results next week or in 2 weeks.

Possible Reactions When Taking Coconut Oil or Virgin Coconut Oil

Some people will experience loose stool or 'feels like diarrhea'. If that happens to you, reduce your daily dosage or split up the intake. Gradually increase the dosage over weeks.

The loose stool is caused by the inability of the digestive system to handle raw oil. This is unlike diarrhea which involves water loss or dehydration.

Some individuals will experience acne flare ups as your body works to clear up your system. I personally experience it for a few weeks. After that it gradually disappeared.

Key Takeaways

- Take Virgin Coconut Oil by the spoonful for up to 3 table spoons
- Replace all cooking oil with coconut oil for better weight loss results
- Take note of certain reactions such as loose stool and flare ups when taking coconut oil

Chapter 6. Celebrities On Coconut Oil Weight Loss
"Relevant Quote or Fact"

I have included this section to lighten the eBook and more for fun than anything else. Personally I am not crazy about whether famous people are using a particular product.

Having said that, I do know there are people who trust their favourite celebrity and therefore tend to follow if the celebrity uses certain products.

Moreover, we need to be certain what we are doing rather than following blindly. Anyway, here it goes...

Dr Oz : Coconut Oil for Faster Metabolism & Weight Loss

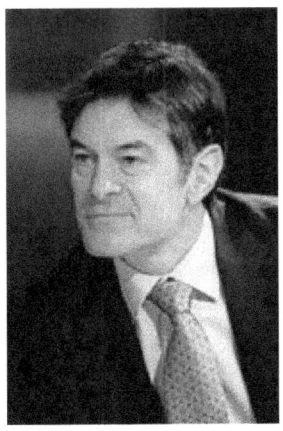

The infamous celebrity doctor, Dr Oz, devoted 2 of his shows to talk about coconut oil.

One of the major benefits Dr Oz talked about on the shows was how coconut oil could speed up the body's metabolism to bring about weight loss.

The shows are very entertaining and if you would like to watch the videos, their links are :
http://www.doctoroz.com/videos/coconut-oil-super-powers-pt-1
http://www.doctoroz.com/videos/coconut-oil-super-powers-pt-2

Jennifer Ashton : Coconut Oil for Weight Loss & Metabolism

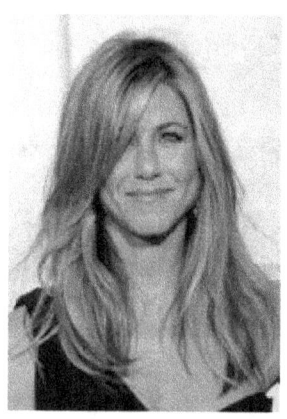

Another superstar whom the press claimed to be on virgin coconut oil is Jennifer Aniston. She was spotted to be shopping with a cart full of coconut oil. Aniston is one of the most commonly cited celebrities to be on coconut oil. Unfortunately I could not trace the source of the information.

Angelina Jolie : Starts Her Day With Virgin Coconut Oil

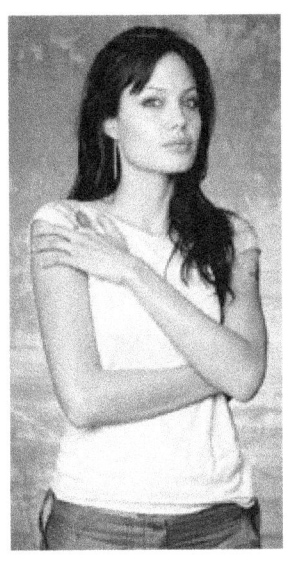

(Jolie's photo source:
http://picasaweb.google.com/lh/photo/MclUe3TBFzHXEL9y1v-rregGRl6j41qDvQWRLSPrsUE)

Angelina Jolie is well known for her slender figure other than her famous lips. According to Stuff.co.nz, "Angelina has been known to start her day with little more than a spoonful of coconut oil and a handful of cereal."

Though she had a double mastectomy in May 2013, she still looks great at 38 (born in 1975). She is known to have a very small appetite and at times she consumes only 600 calories per day. That is probably way below what she should be consuming.

It seems that people around her have been chiding her to eat more but the effort appears to be futile. She has not been able to pack more weight on her 5 feet 7 inch physique!

Miranda Kerr : Consuming Coconut Oil Since She Was 14

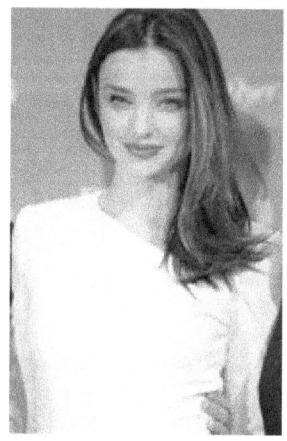

(Photo sources:
http://commons.wikimedia.org/wiki/File:Miranda_Kerr_launches
_new_Qantas_Frequent_Flyer_Rewards_Alliance_-
Sydney%284%29.jpg)

The supermodel from Australia Miranda Kerr says, "I will not go a day without coconut oil. I personally take four tablespoons per day, either on my salads, in my cooking or in my cups of green tea."

If that is true, she has been taking coconut oil for the past 16 years (she is 30 years old).

Gwyneth Paltrow : Slather Her Skin With Coconut Oil

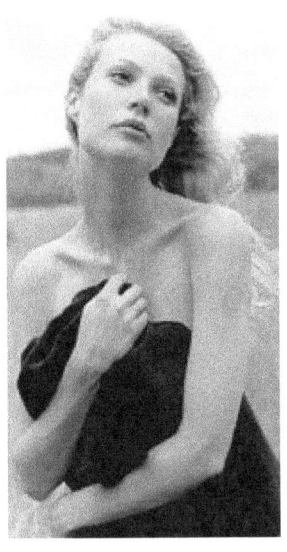

(Photo source:
http://picasaweb.google.com/lh/photo/N9QhZ0pwfrGRB6Ah0yi
S1w)

The Oscar winning actress Gwyneth Paltrow has been reported to use coconut oil on her skin.

A quote from The Healthy Home Economist (<u>visit site here</u>) on Paltrow's use of coconut oil,
"I love Epsom salt baths to detox, revive muscles and de-puff skin. While in the bath, I use an exfoliating mitt which stimulates skin and leaves it soft and bump-free. After the bath, I slather my skin with extra-virgin organic -coconut oil."

There are still other celebrities who are known to utilize coconut oil in their lives. If you are into this, please visit the link below for the 'Top 10 Celebrities Who Use Virgin Coconut Oil':

Key Takeaways

This chapter lists some of the celebrities who are using coconut oil or virgin coconut oil. Regardless of who is using the oil, the most important thing is we ourselves must be sure and convinced of the value and benefits of coconut oil. Do not follow blindly!

Chapter 7. Try Coconut Oil For 3 to 6 Months

Formally, this is the concluding chapter on Coconut Oil Weight Loss. However, I have moved several chapters which were in the original edition of the book to the appendices.

These topics in the appendices will cover related topics on why and when one should lose weight. The concept of true weight loss is also discussed in that section. I would encourage you to read them if you have no idea whether or not you should lose weight. One should definitely be familiarized with true weight loss if he or she is not sure what the body loses in any weight loss program.

Before I make my concluding remarks I would like to thrown in another piece of surprise which 99.99% of the people would not have known.

Is Coconut Oil Still Bad Because It is a Saturated Fat/Oil?

Up until this point in the book, if I have failed to convince you that coconut oil is good, please read the following with full attention (you will be glad you did).

Let us recall the medium-chain fatty acids we discussed in Chapter 2. I showed you a table with a list of fatty acids and their sources. (You can click here to return to that chapter to refresh your memory.)

One of the medium-chain fatty acids in coconut oil is called Lauric acid, a C12 saturated fatty acid. This is one of the most powerful ingredients occurring naturally in coconut oil. The antimicrobial properties of this C12 saturated fatty acid will make your head spin. I will not discuss the fatty acid itself here because my focus is not the details of its antimicrobial power.

Scientists are genetically modifying oil crop to produce more saturated fats!

Remember, this Lauric acid is a 'BAD' **SATURATED** fat according to opponents of coconut oil. If this saturated fat from coconut oil is so **BAD** and **HEALTH DAMAGING**, then why are scientists breeding CANOLA crops to produce HIGHER LAURIC ACID CONTENT? Why would the Canadian Government approve a Genetically-engineered oil crop that produces up to 40% lauric acid, a supposedly BAD SATURATED fat? And, why would the United States allow cultivation of a SATURATED fat producing oil crop for food and for feed?

Yes. This is happening. This has happened! Scientists know very well how powerful this lauric acid is and how this SATURATED fat can benefit our health like no other fatty acids could accomplish. It is so good that they had to GENETICALLY MODIFY and PROGRAM the canola crop so that it can produce lauric acid content, up to 40%. The new breed of canola is called LAURATE CANOLA.

The first Laurate Canola was approved in Canada and planted commercially in 1994. This was covered in 2003 by the Ag Innovation News,

"A DNA-modified canola variety high in laurate, typically found in tropical oils, was first planted commercially by Calgene in 1994."

Source of this news can be viewed here. In 1996 more new breeds of Laurate Canola were approved (source here)

You can find out the details in an article entitled 'Laurate canola looks to be the next oil boom' published back in 1997 by clicking here. You can also find out the detailed database of Laurate Canola here.

Without much elaboration, you can probably conjure up a lot of interpretation of the above information. The intention of those who defamed coconut oil is no longer important or relevant. What is important is the beneficial properties of the saturated fats in coconut oil are so good that they have to be duplicated in other polyunsaturated fat producing crop.

If you started out reading this book with the impression that coconut oil is bad for your health, I hope you rethink the misinformation which has been passed on to you prior to this book. The purpose is not to identify the culprit. The purpose is to re-embrace the unsung greatness of coconut oil.

Final Remarks

I honestly hope you have enjoyed reading this book as much as I have enjoyed putting my thoughts and understanding on this wonderful topic of Coconut Oil and Weight Loss into comprehensible words. I also hope the information contained herein will bring better meaning into your life and health.

My ultimate objective of this book is to dispel the false notion of coconut oil is fattening and bad. I hope I have been able to convey some technical information into something comprehensible for people who has no background in biology, biochemistry or nutrition. I also hope I have been able to persuade those who are contemplating weight loss program to give this wonderful tropical oil a chance to do its work in the body.

Try coconut oil for at least 3 to 6 months. Experience the changes in and on yourself. Any change will likely to be gradual, which I believe is the best way for the body to achieve homeostasis and long term health. Coconut oil is not medicine though it can have medical treatment and healing properties which I hope to address in an upcoming book. Do not expect results to be instant or fast.

Our body development did not take place overnight, in weeks or in months. It took years for an adult body to be developed into its maturity. Our health is also not ruined overnight. In other words, any diseases or most illnesses (other than poisoning and accident) did not happen in days or weeks. Diseases surface after years or decades of abuse. So, it's not fair to expect our body to be rebuilt in days, weeks or even months.

Most people experience something wonderful in taking coconut oil from 3 months onwards. Some people may have it earlier, others later. But it is definitely worth the investment of effort and waiting in time for long term health.

Coconut oil is a large topic as it has many wonderful properties that go beyond weight loss. I am currently working on two other eBooks on coconut oil. One will be on the antimicrobial properties of the oil, while the other will be on its healing properties and diseases.

Download Virgin Coconut Oil and Coconut Oil Overview

Finally, I have done up a sheet which lists the main points on coconut oil and virgin coconut oil. It looks like the following picture which you may or may not be able to view in your Kindle.

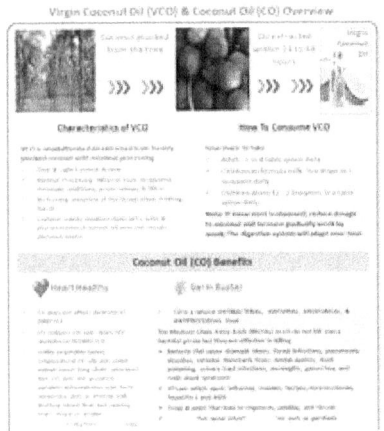

You can download it at http://healthybodytips.org/cowl/. All you need to do is to enter your name and email, and I will email you the download link for the above 'Virgin Coconut Oil and Coconut Oil Overview' as PDF. In the same email, you will also be able to download another pdf 'Diagrams in Coconut Oil WeightLoss' with all the pictures, charts and photos used in the book for those of you who could not view them in their Kindle.

Once again, thank you for purchasing this eBook. If you have any questions or queries, please write to me at jonas@healthybodytips.org. If you are taking coconut oil, I would be honored to know your experience and results.

Oh, by the way, if you have enjoyed reading this book, please do me a great favor in giving your review or sharing by returning to the Kindle store at
http://www.amazon.com/dp/B00E1EV97Y

Your review and sharing will be greatly appreciated.

Take good care of your health. Live healthily!

Jonas Lee

Appendices

Back to Table of Contents

Appendix 1. Should You Lose Weight?

"It's not hard to make decisions when you know what your values are." - Roy Disney

Understanding the reason for losing weight is as important as losing weight itself.
Having a clear reason(s) for losing weight helps us to be focused and makes it easier to reach our weight loss goal. Identifying the right reason for losing weight can help prevent us from unnecessary health consequences.

Why Do People Want To Lose Weight?

People want to lose weight for all kinds of reasons. However, I am of the opinion that not everybody should or needs to lose weight. If your reasons for losing weight are not justifiable or will harm your health in the long run, I urge you to re-consider your intention for shedding weight unnecessarily.

Most weight loss experts agree on the premise that health should be the number one consideration before we take on any weight loss plan. Some weight management plans can bring about quick weight loss results but the consequences can be disastrous down the road.

In Appendix 3, I discuss how our body loses weight. The real dangers with quick weight loss are often tied to jeopardizing the normal functioning of the body.

Once we understand how our body loses weight, we will understand the risks involved when we bring about weight loss beyond the natural limits.

Lose Weight for the Right Reasons without Damaging Your Health

Let's look at some of the common reasons for losing weight.

1. A Great Looking Body

This is the most common reason for people wanting to lose weight. Who doesn't want a great looking body? Everyone wants to have a head-turning figure! There is nothing wrong with that as long as the amount of weight loss does not cause one to be in the underweight zone!

I bet nobody wants a body with fat bouncing up and down around the waist while walking or strolling. This is not to ridicule people who are already in that body condition. We need to realize and accept the hard fact of extra, bouncing fats are not only unsightly but are unhealthy.

Everybody, you and I included, want to have a gorgeous body without any loose fats. That is the most common and natural reason for losing weight.

2. I Don't Want To Be Obese Because I Want To Be Healthy

This is the most justifiable reason for losing weight. When a person is obese (we will look at obesity in the next chapter), it becomes more of a health issue than good looking body. There is no doubt that obesity is a global problem!

Not only more and more adults are overweight, more kids today are overweight and obese. Overweight makes a person more vulnerable to falling ill. Obesity drastically increases the risks of diseases.

If a person is obese, he or she should definitely shed the extra weights for health reasons. I would go as far as saying the need for obese people to lose weight should be immediate. This is because the longer an obese person delays losing weight, the more obese he or she becomes. This happens ten out of ten times. It is a behavioral problem!

If an obese person starts to think that 'I am still OK', he or she will never take action to lose weight. In fact, this is the very psychological and mental sabotage that makes many people overweight and crossing over into the obese zone.

Health should always be the top priority in life. Without health, everything else becomes meaningless. So, losing weight to get out of obesity is not really an option. It is necessary to regain health.

3. I Want To Be Skinny And Have A Supermodel Look!

I personally think that this is one of the most disastrous reasons for wanting to lose weight. Have you known or do you know someone with that kind of goal for their body? Surprisingly, there are many people who think like that.

This is different from no. 1 above. Here, we often witness people who lose weight and end up in the underweight category. Often people who falls into this category end up being anorexic! That is why I believe this reason for losing weight is dangerous.

Being skinny is a very subjective idea or concept. What is considered to be skinny? Skinny means underweight. Though underweight is not as serious a problem as being overweight and obese, it will still get the person into health problems.

How people define being skinny and overweight is also a problem. Sometimes, a person's idea of great body shape can be seriously flawed. It is not easy for the person to admit that.

If you are someone who regard being skinny is great, I hope you reconsider your idea of great looks. Being skinny can get you into serious health problems down the road. You want to be lean but not skinny and underweight. Don't be fooled by the so called 'supermodel' skinny look.

If you are already skinny or underweight, I suggest you lose some 'skinniness' and get back some healthy weight for the sake of your health. You may not feel you are not well if you are still young. But the health disease will come one day if you don't do something about it.

Weight Loss is a Choice

Losing weight is a choice. Hopefully, the choice to lose weight is not due to medical or health problem. The choice to lose weight should be made rationally with the correct justification, on medical or health grounds.

As with anything else in life, sometimes we make the wrong choice based on the wrong idea. Some choices are not so damaging while others can have irreversible consequences. If a choice involves health risks, it is wise to consider and decide carefully and cautiously.

Health consequences can be minor or major. Reversing major health defects can be difficult and frustrating. It can become a very costly affair too.

Key Takeaways

- Lose weight for the right reason, and that reason should always be health or at least with health safety as the top priority
- Losing weight to have a great looking body is fine as long as it doesn't get you into health problems down the road
- Losing weight to be skinnier is a 'no no', especially if you are already skinny
- Losing weight should never harm your health in the long run

Something to Ponder

Do you really want to lose weight? Are you really sure your body is carrying excess weight?

What is the evidence that says you need to lose weight?

The next logical question to address is:

What is the reference weight or number that alerts me to lose weight?
Find out in Appendix 2.

Back to Table of Contents

Appendix 2. When Should You Consider Losing Weight?

" You have to stay in shape. My grandmother, she started walking five miles a day when she was 60. She's 97 today and we don't know where the hell she is." Ellen Degeneres

We have discussed the various reasons for losing weight in Appendix 1. Here we will explore when we should consider losing weight. We need to have some guidelines on whether there really is a need to lose weight.

Here I am referring to the quantifying guidelines, some numbers or indicators. This is critical because if we have no idea at what point we should lose weight, we may simply take on a weight loss program just because we want to or like to!

We really need to know some kind of reference weight range, above or below which we need to consider weight loss or weight gain. So, it is imperative to have an understanding of the guidelines for when we really need to lose weight and when not to lose weight.

Body Weight Classification

The classification of body weight is indicated by what is known as BMI or body mass index. BMI is essentially a number or indicator calculated based on a person's weight and height.

BMI is calculated using the following formula:

BMI=Weight (kg) / Square of Height (m)
Or,
BMI=[Weight (lb) / Square of Height (in)] x 703

If we consider the BMI equation from the view point of logic, it is really an estimation of weight based on our body size. While body sizes will vary from individual to individual, the body systems that produce the body mass should be the same for everyone.

What I mean by that is we all have the same biological structure for our body. However, your body systems and my body systems will differ in many aspects because we have different genetic makeup, dietary habits, etc.

But the weight gaining or losing mechanism should be similar, if not the same, for everybody. That is why scientists are able to come up with some form of guidelines like the BMI index to gauge our expected normal weight.

Though there are controversies on the BMI index, it is a reference. It serves as a guideline for us to know whether or not we are way out of the norm or within the expected average.

BMI Chart

From the above equation, a BMI chart or table can be computed based on weight and height increments. An example of a BMI chart (from British Heart Foundation) is shown below:

For instance, a person with a height of 5 feet 10 inches and a weight of 70 kg would have a BMI of 22, which is in the green zone and therefore is considered normal. (Refer to chart below)

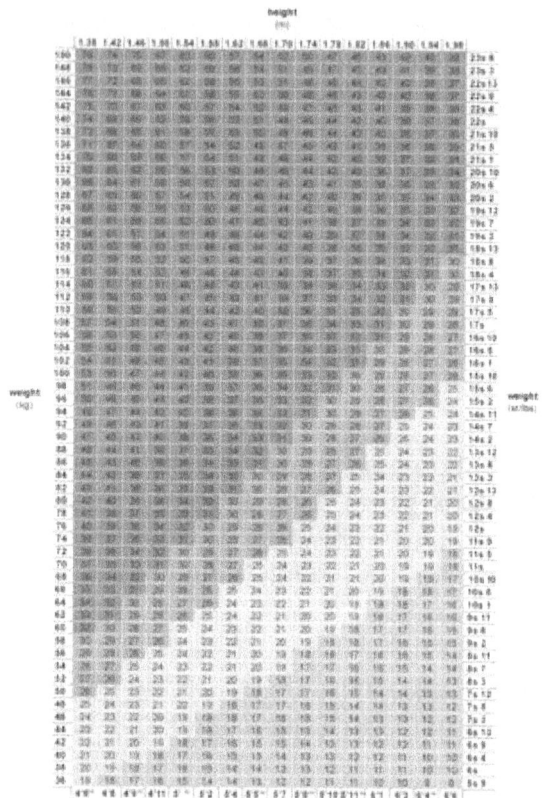

Legend for the chart above, red=obese, orange=overweight, green=normal, blue=underweight.
(Source: BMI Chart. British Heart Foundation.
http://www.bhf.org.uk/bmi/home.html)

If the same person has a weight of 86 kg, he or she would have a BMI of 27, in the orange zone and is deemed to be overweight. If the person's weight is much higher, his or her BMI would be much higher and will fall into the red zone, the obese level. (Refer to chart below)

Guidelines for Obesity, Overweight & Underweight

The interpretation of BMI is summarized in the table below.

BMI	Above 30	25 to 30	18.5 to 25	Below 18.5
Interpretation	Obese	Overweight	Normal	Underweight

WHO's definition for overweight and obesity is the same as defined in the above table. However, there are variations in the ranges depending on the sources of BMI computations.

You might come across certain literature which further categorizes obesity into severe obesity with BMI greater than 35, morbid obesity for BMI above 40, and super obesity for BMI of 45 and above.

BMI may also differ depending on the population types, such as Asian, Caucasians, Chinese, and Japanese. Japanese research scientist Dr Kanazawa and co-workers reported that China defines obesity as BMI greater than 28 while a BMI above 25 is considered obese in Japan.

From the BMI calculations, an index of above 25 is considered to be overweight while underweight is defined as BMI below 18.5. If BMI is above 30, a person is deemed to be obese.

Obesity is Global

According to the March 2013 update by WHO (World Health Organization), there were more than 1.4 billion adults (20 years old and above) overweight in 2008. Out of these 1.4 billion adults, more than 200 million men while close to 300 million women were obese. The update also indicated that more than 40 million children under the age of 5 were overweight in 2011.

The Need To Lose Weight

As you can see, the BMI provides some guidelines on whether we are out of the normal range. When BMI is around the border line, say 26 or 17, the issue is probably not too great to cause worries. However, when our BMI is bordering on 30 or above or way below 18.50, we should do something about our weight rather than ignoring it.

Top 10 Obese Nations in the Developed World

According to **OECD** or *Organisation for Economic Co-operation and Development*'s 2012 updates on obesity rates in its 34 member nations, the top 10 most obese nations are:

1. United States
2. Mexico
3. New Zealand
4. Chile
5. Australia
6. Canada
7. United Kingdom
8. Ireland
9. Luxembourg
10. Finland

Health Risks and Consequences of Obesity

Obesity is really a medical condition that requires treatment before it brings on chronic diseases. More often than not, obese people are already plagued with some of the most common diseases such as Type II diabetes and heart disease.

A recent news on CBS entitled 'Battling American Samoa's 75-percent obesity rate' caught my attention. Apparently, American Samoa island boasts the highest obesity rate of 75% in the world. And that is really high.

According to Dr. John Tuitele, the problems for the island's high obesity are sedentary lifestyles and on islanders' appetite for high-fat American food. Furthermore, Brown University conducted a study which found that 1 in 5 babies on the island are overweight at birth. The scenario gets worse by 15 months, close to 40 percent of boys and 30 percent of girls are overweight or obese.

The source for the above news can be found at http://www.cbsnews.com/8301-18563_162-57592578/battling-american-samoas-75-percent-obesity-rate/.

Research studies have clearly shown that obesity can and will very likely result in illnesses such as cardiovascular diseases, Type II diabetes, sleep disorder, asthma, osteoarthritis, and even cancer. Some of these diseases often result in earlier death than expected. As a result, obesity is said to reduce life expectancy.

Key Takeaways

- Obesity is a global health issue that is becoming increasingly severe.
- A BMI index of 25 and above is considered overweight while 30 and above is considered obese
- Obesity should be taken seriously as it is likely a precursor of many chronic illnesses.
- When a person is obese, he or she should take actions to lose weight immediately
- When a person is overweight, he or she should plan to lose some extra weight soon

Action

- Find out your own BMI if you have never done that before or recently.
- Take stock of your weight condition

Back to Table of Contents

Appendix 3. Weight Loss Explained

"I've been on a diet for two weeks and all I've lost is fourteen days." Totie Fields

The concept of true weight loss is very important. If you get this concept right, you will save yourself a lot of health issues even if you do take up weight loss plan. I have included this discussion is because many people whom I have dealt with relying ONLY on the numbers of the weighing scale as a measure of weight loss. This is very dangerous.

Weight loss is a rather misleading term. Losing weight can mean a lot of things. A drop in number on the weighing scale no doubt indicates weight lost but that reduction could mean much more than just weight drop. It could mean losing fats, water (body fluid), or muscle.

The use of weight loss in our communication does not accurately convey the true meaning of losing unhealthy mass from the body. Fat loss is the better term in place of weight loss. Water loss and muscle loss can have deleterious effects on our body.

In view of the above, we need to have a proper concept and understanding of weight loss. This becomes more critical if you are considering taking up or starting a weight loss program.

You need to make absolutely sure what the end result of a weight loss program is. Will you be losing fats? Or, will you be losing more water and muscle? Do not participate in a program if you are not sure or if the program instructor is not sure.

We often see some advertisements claiming super quick weight loss. Will those programs help you lose weight fast? Absolutely! Can a person lose weight quickly? Certainly! Will you die from going through these programs? Probably not, not so soon anyway.

BUT, you will likely suffer health consequences later on. These advertisements work really well because most of us are impatient and want fast results.

We want quick fix and superfast results. We want overnight cure. We can't wait. Waiting is inefficient. Waiting is no good. But that is exactly how we get into trouble!

What Determine Our Calories Requirements?

Let's start from the basics of the body. We often talk about calories and energy for our body. How does the body handle the energy intake or the calorie requirements?

We eat food for energy which is from the amount of calories in our food. What determines our calorie limit or need? The answer is metabolic rate.

Metabolic Rate - BMR

You might have heard of the term **BMR**. BMR stands for *basal metabolic rate*. BMR tells us how fast our body uses calories for the basic body needs.

That is, when we are inactive and/or lying down during our waking hours, we still burn calories and need energy for basic body needs. The rate of these calories burning or energy production is called BMR

In other words, this is the minimum amount of calories needed to support essential metabolic functions, even when we are not doing anything. The moment we become active or start engaging in activities, even minor activity like walking around the house, we need more than the minimum calories.

It is estimated that at least 60 to 70% of the calories we burn each day is used for basic metabolic functions. Each of us differs in our metabolism. Your BMR and my BMR will be different. Our BMR and the amount of calories we need are determined by many factors.

BMR Differences

Active people burns more calories and hence needs more energy than people who are less active physically. A manual worker requires more calories than a person who sits at the office all day long. An older person will have less calories demand than someone younger.

One shocking fact we seldom hear is an overweight person needs less calories than a person who is more muscular or has a lean body. This is a bad news for overweight or obese people. The reason is overweight or obese people use less calories than lean, muscular people.

It means obese people have to consume even less food in order to have a reduction in weight! That's why when an obese person trying to lose weight without reducing the amount of food intake, his or her chances of losing weight successfully are much lower.

How Do We Gain Weight?

The next logical question to ask is what makes us gain weight? The simple answer is calories. When our body has more calories than it can use or burn, the extra calories must be stored as fats.

The food we eat goes through the processes of digestion and absorption before the calories are converted into energy for our body use. When we consume more food than what we need, the extra calories are preserved as fat storage, which is essentially an energy reservoir. The fat storage consequently makes us gain weight. If there is too much fat storage, we become overweight.

So, How Many Calories Do I Need?

Our daily calorie requirements are determined by the body's basic metabolic functions and also the amount of activity each day. In other words, the amount of physical activities and the amount of food we eat play a role in determining whether we gain weight or lose weight.

There are formulae and charts that tell us the amount of calories we need. We will not be going into the details of these formulae because once we understand the concept behind, we do not need to calculate the exact calories.

Depending on lifestyle and daily activity levels, calorie requirements differ from person to person. For example, a person who weighs about 70kg will need about 1,600 calories to fuel the basic metabolic functions. On top of that the individual will need an additional 1,000 calories per day for normal daily physical activities.

If he or she does additional physical activities such as exercise or jogging, the calorie requirements will increase. If he or she does not replenish those extra calorie needs, he or she will end up burning some of the body fat storage for the extra energy needed.

Increasing physical activity without increasing calorie or food intake will result in weight loss by using the body fats. This is the common method for losing weight.

However, if the person does not exercise or want to exercise, the only options he or she has to lose weight is not to eat, eat less or eat foods with less calories than his or her usual meal.

Sources of Weight Loss – What Are We Losing?

We must identify in losing weight, from where or what our body loses. There are essentially 3 major sources of weight loss, namely, loss of body fluid, muscle loss and fat loss.

(a) Weight Loss – Loss of Body Fluid

This is a very important topic we must discuss when we talk about weight loss. We all know, or most of us know, about 70% of our body is water (or more correctly, fluid). This is a huge amount of water!

When a person loses water, it will result in weight loss. But this is not the kind of weight loss we want because loss of water or fluid from the body can have far deeper problems than we can feel or notice in the short run.

Dehydration

Sometimes, loss of water is used interchangeably with dehydration. Strictly speaking, this is not quite correct. Dehydration is defined medically as excessive loss of body fluid.

Dehydration is a very technical and scientific subject. For instance, hypotonic dehydration refers to loss of electrolytes, especially sodium, from the body. If we really want to understand the health effects of dehydration, one can write volumes of books on this subject.

Effects of Water Loss

Loss of water from the body affects its metabolic processes. This can be serious or mild depending on the amount of water lost. Most of us do not realize we are losing water because we are not aware of the symptoms.

For instance, symptoms for loss of 1% to 2% water from the body may include thirst, mouth dryness, reduced urine volume, dark and cloudy urine, dizziness, fever, tearless cry, headache, tiredness, increased irritability, and more. When the body loses more water, more severe symptoms start to kick in.

When we say loss of water from our body, what do we mean? Where does the water come from? And, how do we lose the water?

Water Loss from Cells

The water really comes from the cells. In other words, water is pulled out of the cells and escaped from the body through breath, sweat, urine and stool. When our cell loses water, it will affect many of the cellular functions.

Disturbance in cellular activities will in turn affect many of the body systems. The wide range of symptoms is really an indication of the water loss chain effects in the body causing imbalances, which if not restored will bring about more severe and deeper damages.

So, stay away from weight loss program that makes you lose body fluids as part of the weight loss process.

(b) Weight Loss – Muscle Loss?

Muscle loss is something we need to mention briefly because it can be an outcome of weight loss program gone awry. This can be much more severe than water loss. The health consequences of muscle loss can land a person into deep health problems which require medical attention.

When there is loss of muscle, the body is likely severely lacking in amino acids, or amino acid deficiency. When this happens for too long, the person may need to undertake amino acid therapy.

Muscle loss is highly likely to occur when weight loss happens too fast. So, beware of programs that promise superfast weight loss! Muscle loss during any weight loss regime will likely be caused by a combination of lack of exercise while dieting.

In other words, a person goes on a diet schedule with too little calorie intake while not doing any exercise at the same time. This type of program is trying to maximize and accelerate weight loss without considering the integrity of the person's health. But this type of program will produce greater and faster weight loss!

What has been observed universally with this type of program is 'one loses weight fast, one also gains back the weight fast!' In other words, the individual ends up in square one again!

In many cases, the person actually gains more weight during the regaining phase. In essence, the weight loss cycle goes through a loop where a person loses weight fast, he or she then packs more weight to the body.

The person who has experienced fast and significant weight loss with the program is likely to go for another round of the program, hoping that the second round will bring lasting result. Then the cycle happens again.

When this lose-weight-gain-weight cycle gets repeated too many times, the body will gradually break down and can no longer sustain the deleterious effects of muscle loss (also water loss).

Remember, muscle loss is something you must avoid at all cost with or without any weight loss program.

(c) True Weight Loss – Fat Loss

Fat loss is really what we should be after if we want or need to lose weight healthily. Losing fat not only fulfills the objective of true weight loss, but also improves our health. I strongly advocate this is the only type of program any person should consider taking up for losing weight.

How Much Fat Can We Lose?

Assuming we want to lose weight by getting rid of the extra fats, how much weight can we lose in reality?

It is generally agreed that one pound of body fat is worth 3,500 calories. So, if you want to lose 1lb of fat, you need to reduce your calorie intake by 3,500 calories. If you want to lose 2 lbs of fat, you need decrease caloric intake by 7,000.

Fat Loss Example

Using our previous example of a 70kg (~150 lb) office worker who needs 1,600 calories for basic metabolic functions plus another 1000 calories for normal daily activity, let us analyze the fat loss possibility.

Let's call this person Jack. Jack has a calorie requirement of about 2,600 per day (based on the above assumption). If Jack wants to lose 1lb of fat, he will need to split up the reduction of his calories intake over a number of days.

In other words, he needs to split the 3,500 calories into several days and reduce the amount of intake accordingly. If he tries to reduce 3,500 calories within 1 to 2 days, he will not have enough calories to perform daily physical activities and handle the basic metabolic functions.

So, it is wiser and more realistic for Jack to split up the calorie reduction over a week. Splitting 3,500 calories over 7 days will yield 500 calories per day.

Therefore, Jack has to reduce 500 calories intake per day if he wants to lose 1ib of fat. If he continues the 500 calorie reduction for two weeks in a row, he will lose 2lb in total.

This illustration is to enable you to see what would happen if you really want to lose fat safely and healthily.

However, there are bodybuilders who push beyond the 2 pounds fat loss per week. The 2lb fat loss weekly limit has been accepted and around for a long time. No one really knows for sure how this comes about.

But from the above example, it is not difficult to see how a person of average weight can only lose a maximum of 2lb based on his daily calorie requirements. If a person tries to lose more, he or she will likely be short of calories for basic metabolic functions, which will be damaging to health.

That's why true and healthy weight loss by losing fat requires time and patience. That's how our body works. You can't push it too far.

Weight Loss in Reality

In reality, weight loss will likely be a mixture of water loss and fat loss if done properly. Body fat likely consists of water and muscle as well. If we do not starve the body beyond its basic metabolic needs and wisely supplement with some exercise, the weight loss result will be seen.

We can always replenish the water through drinking more water, which will balance the water loss, thus resulting in regaining some weight (not fat). So, the body weight loss will be gradual but healthy.

It is better to plan for gradual weight loss than rushing it for short term results. Obese people whose health is under threat may need to go through medical procedure to stabilize the condition before daily weight loss program can be implemented.

Weight Loss in Perspective

It is worth emphasizing that weight loss is not just a physical or physiological affair. The problem of being overweight or obesity is often complicated by other factors such as metabolism, genetic factors, or improper dietary habits developed from upbringing or growing up.

Therefore, in order to have long lasting weight loss, or rather to restore optimal weight, it probably requires changing food habit as well as a change in lifestyle.

Key Takeaways

- Our body manages calorie requirements through metabolic rate

- BMR signifies how fast our body converts calories into energy to meet basic metabolic functions.
- Our daily calorie requirements depend on our level of physical activities
- 3 Sources of weight loss : loss of water, muscle loss and fat loss
- Avoid program which promises quick weight loss and those which result in excessive water loss
- Avoid muscle loss at all costs
- Fat loss should be the only long term objective for weight loss
- Long term success in weight loss requires change in food habit as well as behavioral adjustments

Back to Table of Contents

Download Virgin Coconut Oil and Coconut Oil Overview

I have done up a sheet which lists the main points on coconut oil and virgin coconut oil. It looks like the following picture which you may or may not be able to view in your Kindle.

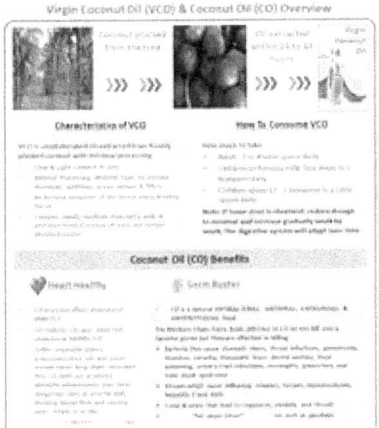

You can download it at http://healthybodytips.org/cowl/. All you need to do is to enter your name and email, and I will email you the download link for the above 'Virgin Coconut Oil and Coconut Oil Overview' as PDF. In the same email, you will also be able to download another pdf 'Diagrams in Coconut Oil WeightLoss' with all the pictures, charts and photos used in the book for those of you who could not view them in their Kindle.

References

1. Obesity and overweight. World Health Organization. Fact sheet N°311, March 2013. (http://www.who.int/mediacentre/factsheets/fs311/en/)
2. Sturm R. Increases in morbid obesity in the USA: 2000–2005. Public Health. 2007 July; 121(7): 492–496 (http://www.ncbi.nlm.nih.gov/pmc/articles/PMC2864630/)
3. Kanazawa M, Yoshiike N, Osaka T, Numba Y, Zimmet P, and Inoue S. Criteria and classification of obesity in Japan and Asia-Oceania. 2002. Asia Pac J Clin Nutr. 11 Suppl 8: S732–S737.
4. http://www.oecd.org/health/49716427.pdf
5. Papamandjaris AA, MacDougall DE, Jones PJ. Medium chain fatty acid metabolism and energy expenditure: obesity treatment implications. Life Sci. 1998;62(14):1203-15.
6. Kanazawa M, Yoshiike N, Osaka T, Numba Y, Zimmet P, and Inoue S. Criteria and classification of obesity in Japan and Asia-Oceania. 2002. Asia Pac J Clin Nutr. 11 Suppl 8: S732–S737.
7. Heidi Skolnik and Andrea Chernus. Nutrient Timing for Peak Performance. 2010. (http://www.humankinetics.com/products/all-products/The-Nutrient-Timing-for-Peak-Performance)
8. Westerterp KR. Diet Induced Thermogenesis. Nutrition & Metabolism 2004, 1:5.
9. Baba, N., Braaco, E.F., Hashim, S.A. 1982. Enhanced thermogenesis and diminished deposition of fat in response to overfeeding with diet containing medium chain triglyceride. American Journal of Clinical Nutrition 35.
10. St-Onge, M-P. and Peter J. H. Jones, P.J.H. 2002. Physiological Effects of Medium-Chain Triglycerides: Potential Agents in the Prevention of Obesity. Journal of Nutrition 132.
11. Hill, J.O., Petersa, J.C., Yanga, D., Sharpa, T., Kalera, M., Abumrada, N.N., Greenea, H.L. 1989.

Thermogenesis in humans during overfeeding with medium-chain triglycerides. In Metabolism. Pp641-648.

12. St-Onge, M-P. and Bosarge, A. 2008. Weight-loss diet that includes consumption of medium-chain triacylglycerol oil leads to a greater rate of weight and fat mass loss than does olive oil. American Journal of Clinical Nutrition 87.

13. Fife, Bruce. 2004. The Coconut Oil Miracle. Avery.

Thank you for purchasing this eBook.

Did you enjoy reading the Book? Or, did you find the information helpful?
I would really appreciate if you would return to the Kindle store and leave a review and rating for this book, because the Kindle rankings are driven by readers and customers like you.

Click or copy this link to your browser to leave a rating for this book:
http://www.amazon.com/dp/B00E1EV97Y

Please take a second to do so if you've enjoyed this book so far.